HIIT WORKOUT FOR ENDOMORPH WOMEN ONLY

Easy Guide to Flexible and Efficient Strength Exercises for Endomorphs.

Jimmy Nicholas

TABLE OF CONTENTS

INTRODUCTION

Welcome, fellow endomorph women adventurers, to a journey that promises to reshape the way you approach fitness and reclaim your power over your body! As we embark on this quest together, armed with sweatbands and determination, let's dive headfirst into the exhilarating world of High-Intensity Interval Training (HIIT) tailored specifically for those of us who proudly wear the endomorph badge.

But first, let's press pause and take a moment to acknowledge the emotions swirling within you. Perhaps you've felt the frustration of trying countless workouts that just don't seem to cater to your unique body type. Maybe you've faced the disheartening cycle of starting a fitness routine with gusto, only to hit a roadblock and find yourself back at square one. Trust me, I've been there, too. And let me tell you, it's about as enjoyable as a root canal on a Monday morning.

But fear not, dear reader, for you are not alone in this endeavor. Picture me as your trusty sidekick, equipped not only with a plethora of fitness knowledge but also armed with empathy as vast as the Grand Canyon. Together, we'll go through the peaks and valleys of the fitness armed with determination, resilience, and just a dash of humor to keep things light.

Now, before we dive headlong into the exhilarating world of sweat and endorphins, let's take a moment to outline our grand adventure ahead. Our journey begins with a gentle introduction to the concept of HIIT, a fitness phenomenon that's been taking the world by storm. But fear not, my friends, for we'll unravel its mysteries together, like a pair of sleuths on the trail of the perfect burpee.

Next on our itinerary is a deep dive into the world of endomorph body types. Ah yes, the infamous "E" word that's been whispered in locker rooms and fitness forums alike. But fear not, my fellow endomorphs, for we shall embrace our unique characteristics with the same fervor that we embrace a post-workout protein shake.

With our understanding of HIIT and endomorphism firmly in place, it's time to explore the symbiotic relationship between the two. Spoiler alert: it's a match made in fitness heaven. From torching calories to sculpting muscles, HIIT has a knack for turning our fitness dreams into sweaty reality.

But wait, there's more! No adventure would be complete without proper preparation, and our journey into the realm of HIIT is no exception. We'll discuss everything from warming up those muscles to ensuring that our workout space is as inviting as a cozy fireplace on a winter's eve.

And what's an adventure without a bit of customization? Fear not, my fellow adventurers, for we'll explore how to tailor our HIIT routines to suit our individual goals, whether we're aiming to shed pounds, sculpt muscles, or simply feel like the badass warriors that we are.

But enough talk, my friends! It's time to roll up our sleeves, lace up our sneakers, and dive headfirst into the exhilarating world of HIIT for endomorph women. So grab your water bottle, crank up the music, and let's embark on this epic journey together. The road ahead may be challenging, but fear not, for with determination, resilience, and just a sprinkle of humor, we'll conquer mountains and leap over obstacles like fitness ninjas on a mission. Let the adventure begin!

Overview of HIIT (High-Intensity Interval Training)

HIIT training stands for High Intensity Interval Training - a form of cardiovascular exercise. HIIT can be further broken down into two main categories SIT (sprint interval training) and HIT (high intensity training). HIIT training is great for those who are short on time as a way of maximizing your time spent in the gym. A typical HIT session, not including your warm up, would last a maximum of 20 minutes. HIIT is a form of cardiovascular exercise that alternates between short bursts of intense activity and brief periods of rest or low-intensity recovery. This ingenious approach not only revs up your heart rate but also ignites your metabolism, sending it into overdrive long after your workout has come to an end. It's like lighting a firecracker under your body's furnace, incinerating calories with every explosive burst of effort.

But the magic of HIIT doesn't stop there. Oh no, my friends, it goes much deeper than a mere calorie burn. You see, when you push your body to its limits during those intense intervals, you're not just sculpting your muscles; you're also triggering a cascade of physiological responses that leave your body stronger, fitter, and more resilient than ever before.

Unlocking the Potential: Why HIIT Works

So, what is it about HIIT that makes it so darn effective? Well, my fellow seekers of fitness truth, the answer lies in its ability to tap into the very essence of human physiology. You see, our bodies are finely tuned machines, capable of remarkable feats of endurance and strength. But all too often, we find ourselves trapped in the monotony of steady-state cardio or endless hours on the elliptical, never truly pushing our limits or unlocking our full potential.

HIIT, however, flips the script on traditional exercise wisdom, challenging our bodies to adapt and evolve in ways we never thought possible. By alternating between high-intensity bursts and periods of rest, we force our muscles to work harder, our hearts to beat faster, and our lungs to gasp for air like never before. And in doing so, we unleash a torrent of growth hormones and endorphins that flood our bodies with energy and vitality, leaving us feeling invigorated and alive.

But perhaps the most beautiful aspect of HIIT lies in its adaptability. Whether you're a seasoned athlete or a newcomer to the world of fitness, HIIT can be tailored to suit your individual needs and abilities. From sprinting on the track to cycling on the stationary bike, the possibilities are as vast as the open sky, limited only by your imagination and willingness to push beyond your comfort zone.

Now, before you lace up your sneakers and dive headfirst into the world of HIIT, it's important to remember that Rome wasn't built in a day, and neither is a sculpted physique. Patience, my friends, is the name of the game, as is a healthy dose of self-compassion and understanding.

Yes, HIIT may be intense. Yes, it may leave you breathless and sweaty and wondering why on earth you signed up for this in the first place. But remember, dear reader, that every drop of sweat, every gasp for air, is a testament to your commitment to yourself and your health. So, embrace the burn, relish the challenge, and know that with every step, you're one step closer to unlocking the best version of yourself.

Explanation of Endomorph Body Type

Endomorph describes a body type that is characterized by a shorter stature with a wide frame and a higher body fat composition. Typically, endomorphs can easily put on muscle mass, but they also have a slower metabolism, higher fat percentage, and have more difficulty with weight loss. Endomorphs have softer bodies with curves. They have a wide waist and hips and large bones, though they may or may not be overweight. Their weight is often in their hips, thighs, and lower abdomen. Endomorphs often have lots of body fat and muscle and tend to gain weight easily. Many people are combination endomorphs, with delicate upper bodies and fat storage in the midsection or hips and thighs. Endomorphs have narrow shoulders and fat deposits in the lower abdomen, hips, and thighs. This distribution of body weight and fat makes it challenging to reduce weight and needs precise training methods. Of course, you must combine these with a suitable diet to lose weight. Exercise is crucial for endomorphs. It helps build muscle and enhance metabolism. The endomorph somatotype comes with a slower metabolism and additional fat. You must commit to a lifelong exercise plan to achieve and sustain lean body mass. Endomorphs are also well-adjusted emotionally and psychologically, being social, emotionally stable, extroverted, easy to communicate with, and courteous to others.

You can't change the body type you were born with, but you can certainly make it the best it can be. You can increase muscle mass and reduce body fat. A good workout plan will improve strength, endurance, and skills. The slow metabolism associated with the endomorph body type often results from sedentary habits and long-term positive calorie balance. Your resolve and capable guidance can change both your habits and your health. Diligence and consistency go a long way in achieving good health and a desirable body shape.

CHAPTER 1
UNDERSTANDING ENDOMORPH BODY TYPE

Characteristics of Endomorphs

Among various physiques, the endomorph stands out as a testament to the beauty of resilience and strength. Join me on a journey of exploration as we delve into the characteristics that define the endomorph body type and uncover the secrets to embracing our unique physiques with pride and confidence.

The Endomorph: An Introduction to the Body Type

Let's begin by painting a picture of the endomorph physique. Imagine a figure with softer, rounder contours, characterized by a tendency to store excess weight, particularly around the midsection. This genetic predisposition often leads to a fuller, more curvaceous appearance, reminiscent of classic beauty ideals throughout history. But beyond the surface lies a deeper truth: the endomorph body type is not a limitation, but rather a unique expression of genetic diversity. It is a testament to the incredible adaptability of the human body and the power of resilience in the face of adversity.

Strength in Softness: Exploring the Unique Traits of Endomorphs

One of the defining characteristics of the endomorph body type is its innate strength and resilience. Despite the challenges of carrying excess weight, endomorphs possess a remarkable capacity for endurance and stamina. Whether tackling a grueling workout or navigating the ups and downs of daily life, endomorphs rise to the occasion with grace and determination.

Additionally, endomorphs often exhibit a natural athleticism and muscularity that belies their softer exterior. While they may not possess the lean, sculpted physique of their ectomorph counterparts, endomorphs excel in activities that require power, strength, and agility.

The Weighty Issue: Addressing Challenges with Compassion and Understanding

Of course, it would be remiss to discuss the characteristics of endomorphs without acknowledging the challenges they may face in maintaining a healthy weight. The tendency to store excess fat can lead to frustration and self-doubt, particularly in a society that prizes thinness above all else.

But let us pause for a moment of reflection. Instead of viewing excess weight as a failure or a flaw, let us recognize it for what it truly is: a natural variation in body size and shape. It is not a reflection of worth or value, but simply a part of who we are as individuals.

Finding Balance: Nurturing Body and Soul

In the pursuit of health and happiness, it is important for endomorphs to focus not only on physical fitness, but also on nurturing their mental and emotional well-being. Practices such as mindfulness, self-care, and self-compassion can help endomorphs cultivate a positive body image and embrace their unique physiques with love and acceptance.

Additionally, finding a balance between nutrition and exercise is key to maintaining a healthy weight and supporting overall well-being. By focusing on nourishing foods and engaging in regular physical activity that brings joy and fulfillment, endomorphs can cultivate a lifestyle that supports their unique needs and goals.

Challenges and Advantages for Endomorph Women in Fitness

The journey towards fitness can be a daunting one, filled with pitfalls and setbacks that threaten to derail even the most determined of souls. Join me as we explore the challenges that endomorph women face in their pursuit of fitness, and uncover the strategies for overcoming these obstacles with grace and resilience.

The Weight of Expectations: Society's Ideal Body Image

One of the most pervasive challenges for endomorph women in fitness is the pressure to conform to society's idealized standards of beauty and thinness. From glossy magazine covers to airbrushed Instagram feeds, we are bombarded with images of slender, toned bodies that seem to represent the pinnacle of health and desirability. But let us pause for a moment of reflection. The truth is, beauty comes in all shapes and sizes, and there is no one-size-fits-all definition of health and fitness. Instead of striving to attain an unrealistic ideal, let us celebrate the diversity of the human body and embrace our unique physiques with love and acceptance.

The Battle of the Bulge: Struggling to Shed Excess Weight

For endomorph women, the battle of the bulge can feel like an uphill climb with no end in sight. Despite their best efforts, they may find themselves struggling to shed excess weight, particularly around the midsection. This can lead to feelings of frustration, self-doubt, and even shame, as they compare themselves to others who seem to effortlessly maintain a lean, toned physique.

But let us reframe the narrative. Instead of viewing weight loss as the ultimate measure of success, let us focus on cultivating a healthy lifestyle that nourishes our bodies and supports our overall well-being. By making small, sustainable changes to our diet and exercise habits, we can create a foundation for long-term health and vitality, regardless of the number on the scale.

The Perils of Comparison: Overcoming Self-Doubt and Insecurity

In today's hyper-connected world, it's all too easy to fall into the trap of comparison, measuring our worth against the seemingly flawless lives of others. For endomorph women, this can be particularly challenging, as they may feel like they don't measure up to the unrealistic standards set by society.

But let us remember that comparison is the thief of joy, and true happiness comes from within. Instead of fixating on what we perceive as flaws or shortcomings, let us celebrate our strengths and accomplishments, no matter how small they may seem. By cultivating a mindset of gratitude and self-compassion, we can free ourselves from the shackles of comparison and embrace our unique journey towards health and fitness.

Advantages for Endomorph Women.

What if I told you that beneath those soft curves lies a hidden reservoir of strength and resilience, waiting to be unleashed? Join me as we explore the unique advantages that endomorph women bring to the table in their journey towards health and fitness, and discover how embracing their natural gifts can lead to empowerment and success.

Endurance and Stamina: The Secret Weapons of Endomorphs

One of the most notable advantages of endomorph women in fitness is their remarkable endurance and stamina. While others may tire quickly or struggle to maintain intensity during workouts, endomorphs have the ability to push through even the toughest of challenges with grace and determination. Whether it's tackling a high-intensity interval training session or conquering a long-distance run, endomorph women excel in activities that require sustained effort and resilience.

Strength and Power: Harnessing the Power Within

Another advantage of endomorph women in fitness is their natural strength and power. Despite their softer appearance, endomorphs possess a strong, muscular physique that is well-suited to activities that require explosive strength and agility. From lifting weights to sprinting on the track, endomorph women have the ability to excel in a wide range of physical pursuits, making them formidable competitors in the world of fitness.

Natural Resilience: Bouncing Back from Setbacks

Perhaps one of the most underrated advantages of endomorph women in fitness is their natural resilience. Endomorphs are no strangers to setbacks and challenges, but instead of letting these obstacles defeat them, they use them as opportunities for growth and self-improvement. Whether it's a plateau in weight loss or a nagging injury, endomorph women have the ability to bounce back stronger and more determined than ever before, turning adversity into triumph with each step of their journey.

Adaptability: Flexibility in Fitness

Endomorph women also possess a unique ability to adapt to a variety of fitness modalities and training styles. Whether it's yoga, Pilates, CrossFit, or dance, endomorphs thrive in environments that challenge both their minds and bodies, embracing the diversity of movement and expression that each discipline offers. This adaptability not only keeps workouts interesting and engaging but also ensures that endomorph women are constantly challenging themselves and pushing their limits in pursuit of their fitness goals.

Self-Compassion and Acceptance: Embracing the Journey

Finally, one of the greatest advantages of endomorph women in fitness is their capacity for self-compassion and acceptance. Instead of striving for unrealistic ideals or beating themselves up over perceived flaws, endomorphs approach their fitness journey with a sense of grace and humility, recognizing that true health and happiness come from within. By embracing their bodies and celebrating their unique strengths and abilities, endomorph women inspire others to do the same, creating a ripple effect of empowerment and self-love in the world of fitness and beyond.

CHAPTER 2
BENEFITS OF HIIT FOR ENDOMORPH WOMEN

Fat Loss and Metabolic Boost

From glossy magazine covers to late-night infomercials, we're bombarded with promises of quick fixes and miracle cures that claim to melt away the pounds and rev up our metabolism in the blink of an eye. But amidst the noise and confusion, it can be easy to lose sight of the science behind these claims and the strategies that actually work. Join me as we unravel the mysteries of fat loss and metabolic boost, and discover how to harness their power to achieve lasting health and wellness.

The Skinny on Fat Loss: Understanding the Basics

Let's start by demystifying the concept of fat loss. At its core, fat loss is simply a matter of creating a calorie deficit, whereby you consume fewer calories than you expend through daily activities and exercise. This forces your body to tap into its fat stores for energy, resulting in a gradual reduction in body fat over time.

But here's the catch: not all calories are created equal. While it's true that creating a calorie deficit is essential for fat loss, the quality of the calories you consume also plays a crucial role in determining your success. Focusing on nutrient-dense, whole foods such as fruits, vegetables, lean proteins, and healthy fats can help support fat loss while providing your body with the essential nutrients it needs to thrive.

Supercharging Your Metabolism: Separating Fact from Fiction
Next, let's tackle the elusive concept of metabolic boost. Your metabolism, often likened to a furnace that burns calories for energy, is a complex system of biochemical processes that regulate energy expenditure and nutrient metabolism in the body. While some people seem to have a naturally fast metabolism, others may struggle to rev up their metabolic rate, leading to frustration and despair.

But fear not, dear reader, for there are strategies you can employ to supercharge your metabolism and optimize fat loss. One of the most effective ways to boost your metabolism is through regular exercise, particularly high-intensity interval training (HIIT), which has been shown to increase metabolic rate both during and after exercise.

In addition to exercise, incorporating strength training into your routine can also help increase lean muscle mass, which in turn can boost your resting metabolic rate and support fat loss. And let's not forget the power of protein, which has been shown to increase metabolism through a process known as the thermic effect of food, whereby your body burns more calories digesting protein than it does digesting carbohydrates or fats.

Mind over Matter: The Role of Mindfulness in Fat Loss

Finally, let's not overlook the importance of mindset when it comes to fat loss and metabolic boost. In a world obsessed with quick fixes and instant gratification, it can be easy to fall into the trap of unrealistic expectations and self-sabotaging behaviors. But true fat loss and metabolic boost require patience, consistency, and a healthy dose of self-compassion.

Instead of focusing solely on the number on the scale, shift your attention to how you feel both physically and emotionally. Celebrate the small victories along the way, whether it's lifting a heavier weight in the gym or choosing a nourishing meal over a sugary treat. By cultivating a mindset of gratitude and self-compassion, you'll not only support your fat loss and metabolic goals but also create a sustainable foundation for lifelong health and wellness.

Improved Cardiovascular Health

Every aspect of our being depends on the proper functioning of this complex network of arteries, veins, and capillaries. Join me as we delve into the importance of improved cardiovascular health, and discover the transformative impact it can have on our overall well-being.

The Heart of the Matter: Understanding Cardiovascular Health

Let's start by unraveling the mysteries of cardiovascular health. At its core, cardiovascular health refers to the ability of the heart and blood vessels to function efficiently and effectively, delivering oxygen-rich blood to every cell and tissue in the body. But achieving and maintaining optimal cardiovascular health requires more than just a strong heartbeat; it requires a holistic approach that encompasses lifestyle factors such as diet, exercise, and stress management.

Pumping Up the Volume: The Benefits of Improved Cardiovascular Health

So, what exactly are the benefits of improved cardiovascular health? Well, dear reader, the list is long and impressive. From reduced risk of heart disease and stroke to improved circulation and energy levels, the benefits of a healthy heart extend far beyond the confines of our chests. But perhaps the most profound benefit of all is the gift of longevity, allowing us to live longer, healthier lives filled with vitality and purpose.

Getting to the Heart of the Matter: Strategies for Improving Cardiovascular Health

Now that we understand the importance of improved cardiovascular health, let's explore some strategies for achieving this lofty goal. First and foremost, regular physical activity is key. Whether it's brisk walking, jogging, swimming, or cycling, engaging in aerobic exercise strengthens the heart muscle, improves circulation, and lowers blood pressure, reducing the risk of heart disease and stroke. In addition to exercise, maintaining a healthy diet is essential for cardiovascular health. Emphasizing whole foods such as fruits, vegetables, lean proteins, and whole grains while minimizing processed foods, saturated fats, and added sugars can help support heart health and lower cholesterol levels.

Matters of the Heart: The Role of Stress Management and Mental Well-Being

But let us not overlook the importance of stress management and mental well-being in the quest for improved cardiovascular health. Chronic stress, anxiety, and depression can take a toll on the heart, increasing the risk of heart disease and other cardiovascular conditions. By practicing relaxation techniques such as deep breathing, meditation, and yoga, we can calm the mind, soothe the spirit, and protect the heart from the damaging effects of stress.

Muscle Tone and Strength

From the graceful sweep of a dancer's limbs to the powerful thrust of an athlete's sprint, every movement we make is a testament to the strength and resilience of these incredible fibers. Join me as we explore the importance of muscle tone and strength, and discover how harnessing their power can lead to a lifetime of health, vitality, and well-being.

The Building Blocks of Strength: Understanding Muscle Tone and Strength

Let's start by demystifying the concept of muscle tone and strength. At its core, muscle tone refers to the level of tension or contraction present in a muscle at rest, while muscle strength refers to the maximum force that a muscle can generate during contraction. Together, these two components form the foundation of our physical strength and functional capacity, allowing us to perform everyday tasks with ease and grace.

The Benefits of Muscle Tone and Strength: More Than Meets the Eye

But the benefits of muscle tone and strength extend far beyond the realm of physical appearance. While it's true that well-defined muscles can enhance our aesthetic appeal and boost our confidence, the true value of muscle tone and strength lies in their ability to support our overall health and well-being. From improved posture and balance to enhanced metabolism and bone density, strong muscles are the unsung heroes of longevity and vitality.

Building Muscle: The Key to Unlocking Your Potential

So, how exactly do we build muscle tone and strength? The answer, dear reader, lies in the time-tested principles of resistance training and progressive overload. By challenging our muscles with progressively heavier weights or resistance bands, we stimulate muscle growth and adaptation, leading to increases in both muscle tone and strength over time.

But here's the catch: building muscle takes time, patience, and consistency. It's not something that happens overnight, nor is it something that can be achieved with a quick fix or miracle pill. Instead, it requires dedication, hard work, and a commitment to pushing past our limits and challenging ourselves to grow stronger with each passing day.

Functional Fitness: Beyond the Mirror

But let us not forget the importance of functional fitness in our quest for muscle tone and strength. While it's tempting to focus solely on sculpting our bodies for aesthetic purposes, true strength lies in our ability to move with grace and efficiency in our everyday lives. Whether it's lifting groceries, playing with our children, or climbing a flight of stairs, strong muscles are the foundation of functional fitness, allowing us to navigate the challenges of daily life with confidence and ease.

CHAPTER 3
PREPARING FOR YOUR HIIT WORKOUT

Consultation with a Healthcare Professional

It's easy to get lost in a sea of conflicting advice and opinions. But fear not, dear reader, for there is a guiding light that can help illuminate the path forward: consultation with a healthcare professional. Join me as we explore the importance of seeking guidance from a trusted healthcare provider, and discover how their expertise can empower you to take control of your health and well-being.

The First Step: Setting the Stage for Success

Let's start by acknowledging the importance of consultation with a healthcare professional as the first step on your health journey. Whether you're looking to lose weight, manage a chronic condition, or simply improve your overall well-being, a healthcare provider can help assess your current health status, identify any potential risk factors or underlying health issues, and develop a personalized plan to help you achieve your goals.

A Holistic Approach: Beyond the Symptoms

But consultation with a healthcare professional is about more than just addressing your immediate health concerns; it's about taking a holistic approach to your well-being. Unlike the quick-fix solutions offered by fad diets and trendy wellness trends, healthcare professionals take the time to consider the full spectrum of factors that contribute to your health, including your medical history, lifestyle habits, and emotional well-being.

By taking a comprehensive view of your health, healthcare professionals can help you identify and address the root causes of your health issues, rather than simply treating the symptoms. This holistic approach not only leads to more effective outcomes but also empowers you to take ownership of your health and make informed decisions that will benefit you for years to come.

A Source of Expertise and Guidance: Leveraging the Power of Knowledge

In addition to their holistic approach, healthcare professionals also bring a wealth of knowledge and expertise to the table. With years of training and experience under their belts, they have the skills and insights necessary to interpret complex medical information.

Whether it's explaining the latest research findings, interpreting lab results, or guiding you through the maze of treatment options, healthcare professionals serve as invaluable sources of information and support on your health journey. By leveraging their expertise, you can gain a deeper understanding of your health and make informed decisions that align with your goals and values.

A Trusted Partner: Building a Relationship Based on Trust and Respect

But perhaps most importantly, consultation with a healthcare professional is about building a relationship based on trust and respect. Unlike the impersonal interactions often found in the healthcare system, a trusted healthcare provider takes the time to listen to your concerns, validate your experiences, and partner with you to develop a plan of action that meets your unique needs and preferences.

By fostering a supportive and collaborative relationship with your healthcare provider, you can feel confident knowing that you have a trusted ally by your side as you navigate the ups and downs of your health journey. Whether it's celebrating your successes, addressing your concerns, or providing a shoulder to lean on during difficult times, your healthcare provider is there to support you every step of the way.

Equipment and Space Requirements

Before diving into the world of equipment and space requirements, it's important to take a moment to reflect on your fitness goals and aspirations. Are you looking to build strength and muscle tone? Improve cardiovascular health? Enhance flexibility and mobility? By clarifying your objectives, you can better determine the types of equipment and space needed to support your journey.

Quality Over Quantity: Choosing the Right Equipment

When it comes to selecting fitness equipment, quality reigns supreme. While it may be tempting to fill your space with a multitude of gadgets and gizmos, it's far more effective to invest in a few high-quality pieces that align with your goals and preferences. Whether it's dumbbells, resistance bands, kettlebells, or a yoga mat, choose equipment that is versatile, durable, and well-suited to your needs.

But remember, dear reader, that you don't need fancy equipment to get fit. Bodyweight exercises such as squats, lunges, push-ups, and planks can be incredibly effective for building strength and improving fitness, requiring nothing more than your own body and a small space to move.

Making Room for Movement: Creating Your Fitness Space

Once you've chosen your equipment, it's time to carve out a dedicated space for your fitness endeavors. Ideally, this space should be quiet, well-lit, and free from distractions, allowing you to focus fully on your workouts and achieve maximum results. Whether it's a spare room, a corner of your living room, or a section of your backyard, find a space that feels comfortable and inviting, and make it your own.

Consider investing in a few key elements to enhance your fitness space, such as a full-length mirror to check your form, a Bluetooth speaker to pump up the jams, and perhaps a plant or two to add a touch of greenery and inspiration. Remember, dear reader, that your fitness space is a reflection of your commitment to yourself and your health, so make it a place that brings you joy and motivation.

Maximizing Your Resources: Creative Solutions for Limited Space

But what if space is limited, you ask? Fear not, for where there's a will, there's a way. With a bit of creativity and ingenuity, you can transform even the tiniest of spaces into a functional fitness haven. Consider using multi-purpose furniture such as a sturdy coffee table or ottoman for step-ups or tricep dips, or utilizing household items such as towels, cans of food, or water bottles as makeshift weights. You can also take advantage of outdoor spaces such as parks, trails, or playgrounds for your workouts, soaking up the fresh air and sunshine while you sweat. And don't forget the power of virtual fitness classes and online workouts, which allow you to exercise in the comfort of your own home with minimal equipment and space requirements.

Warm-up and Safety Considerations

With a unique body type that tends to store more fat and build muscle at a slower rate, it's essential to approach exercise with care and consideration. Join me as we explore the importance of warm-up and safety considerations for endomorphs, and discover how taking the time to prepare your body can help you achieve your fitness goals safely and effectively.

The Power of Preparation: Understanding the Warm-up

Let's start by diving into the world of warm-ups. Often overlooked or rushed through in the eagerness to get to the main event, warm-ups play a crucial role in preparing your body for exercise. By gradually increasing your heart rate, loosening your muscles, and lubricating your joints, a proper warm-up helps reduce the risk of injury and improve performance during your workout.

For endomorphs, who may be more prone to joint stiffness and mobility issues, a thorough warm-up is especially important. Consider incorporating dynamic stretches, such as arm circles, leg swings, and hip circles, to gently mobilize your joints and increase blood flow to your muscles. This will help prepare your body for the demands of exercise and ensure that you can move with ease and grace throughout your workout.

Safety First: Considerations for Endomorphs

In addition to warming up properly, it's also important for endomorphs to consider safety precautions when engaging in exercise. Due to their larger body size and potential joint issues, endomorphs may be more susceptible to certain types of injuries, such as strains, sprains, and overuse injuries. Therefore, it's essential to approach exercise with caution and listen to your body's signals to avoid pushing yourself too hard or too fast.

When choosing exercises, opt for low-impact activities that are gentle on the joints, such as walking, swimming, cycling, or yoga. These activities not only provide an effective workout but also reduce the risk of injury and allow you to build strength and endurance gradually over time. And don't forget to listen to your body and modify exercises as needed to accommodate any physical limitations or discomfort.

Mindful Movement: Cultivating Body Awareness

Beyond the physical aspects of warm-up and safety considerations, it's also important for endomorphs to cultivate a sense of body awareness and mindfulness during exercise. Pay attention to how your body feels as you move, and honor its signals and limitations with kindness and compassion. If something doesn't feel right, don't push through the pain; instead, modify the exercise or seek guidance from a qualified fitness professional.

By approaching exercise with mindfulness and self-compassion, you can create a safe and supportive environment for your body to thrive. Remember that progress is not measured by how hard or fast you push yourself, but by how well you listen to your body and honor its needs. So take your time, be patient with yourself, and trust that with consistency and dedication, you will achieve your fitness goals in a safe and sustainable way.

CHAPTER 4
CUSTOMIZING HIIT FOR ENDOMORPH WOMEN

Adaptations for Body Composition Goals

With a body type predisposed to storing fat and building muscle at a slower rate, achieving your body composition goals may require a unique approach. Join me as we explore the adaptations tailored specifically for endomorphs, empowering you to unlock your full potential and achieve the body of your dreams with confidence and grace.

Understanding Endomorphs: Embracing Your Unique Body Type

Before diving into the adaptations for body composition goals, it's essential to understand what sets endomorphs apart. Endomorphs typically have a rounder or softer appearance, with a tendency to store fat in areas such as the abdomen, hips, and thighs. While this may present challenges in achieving a lean physique, it's important to recognize that endomorphs also have unique strengths, such as strong bones and a natural propensity for gaining muscle.

Nutrition: Fueling Your Body for Success

One of the key adaptations for endomorphs seeking to optimize their body composition is nutrition. With a slower metabolism and a tendency to store fat more readily, endomorphs may benefit from a diet that focuses on balancing macronutrients and controlling portion sizes. Emphasizing whole, nutrient-dense foods such as lean proteins, fruits, vegetables, and healthy fats can help support fat loss while preserving muscle mass.

Additionally, paying attention to meal timing and distribution throughout the day can help regulate blood sugar levels and prevent overeating. Consider spacing your meals and snacks evenly throughout the day to keep hunger and cravings at bay and maintain stable energy levels.

Exercise: Tailoring Your Workout Routine

When it comes to exercise, endomorphs may need to tailor their workout routines to support their body composition goals. While any form of physical activity is beneficial, incorporating a combination of strength training and cardiovascular exercise can help maximize fat loss and build lean muscle mass.

Strength training, in particular, is essential for endomorphs looking to transform their body composition. Focus on compound movements that target multiple muscle groups simultaneously, such as squats, deadlifts, lunges, and push-ups. These exercises not only burn calories during your workout but also increase muscle mass, which in turn boosts your metabolism and supports fat loss over time.

In addition to strength training, incorporating cardiovascular exercise into your routine can help increase calorie expenditure and improve cardiovascular health. Aim for a mix of high-intensity interval training (HIIT) and steady-state cardio to maximize fat burning and optimize your body composition.

Rest and Recovery: Listening to Your Body

Finally, let's not overlook the importance of rest and recovery in the quest for optimal body composition. Endomorphs may need to pay extra attention to their recovery strategies to avoid burnout and support their body's natural healing processes. Make sure to prioritize quality sleep, as inadequate sleep can disrupt hormone levels and hinder fat loss efforts.

Additionally, incorporating rest days into your workout routine is essential for preventing overtraining and allowing your muscles to repair and grow. Listen to your body's signals and adjust your training intensity and frequency accordingly to ensure that you're striking the right balance between effort and recovery.

Modifications for Joint Health and Comfort

Endomorphs may be more susceptible to joint pain and discomfort during exercise. Join me as we explore the modifications tailored specifically for endomorphs to support joint health and comfort, empowering you to move with ease and grace on your fitness journey.

Understanding Endomorphs: Recognizing Your Unique Needs

Before delving into the modifications for joint health and comfort, it's essential to understand the unique characteristics of endomorphs. Endomorphs typically have a larger body size and a higher percentage of body fat, which can put added strain on the joints, particularly weight-bearing joints such as the knees, hips, and ankles. Additionally, endomorphs may experience reduced mobility and flexibility, making certain exercises and movements more challenging.

Choosing the Right Activities: Low-Impact Exercise Options

One of the key modifications for joint health and comfort for endomorphs is choosing the right activities. While high-impact exercises such as running and jumping may be too harsh on the joints, there are plenty of low-impact options that provide an effective workout without exacerbating joint pain. Consider incorporating activities such as walking, swimming, cycling, or using an elliptical machine, which are gentler on the joints while still providing cardiovascular and strength benefits.

In addition to low-impact cardio, endomorphs may also benefit from incorporating activities that focus on mobility and flexibility, such as yoga, Pilates, or tai chi. These exercises help improve joint range of motion, reduce stiffness, and enhance overall flexibility, making them ideal for supporting joint health and comfort.

Proper Form and Technique: Ensuring Safe Movement Patterns

Another important modification for joint health and comfort for endomorphs is paying attention to proper form and technique during exercise. Poor alignment and technique can put added stress on the joints and increase the risk of injury, particularly for those with larger body sizes. Take the time to learn correct movement patterns and cues for each exercise, and focus on maintaining good posture and alignment throughout your workout.

If you're unsure about proper form, consider working with a qualified fitness professional who can provide guidance and support. They can help you modify exercises as needed to accommodate your body size and mobility limitations, ensuring that you're moving safely and effectively.

Listening to Your Body: Honoring Your Limits

Above all, it's essential for endomorphs to listen to their bodies and honor their limits when it comes to exercise. Pay attention to any signs of discomfort or pain during workouts, and adjust your intensity or modify exercises as needed to avoid exacerbating joint issues. Remember that progress is not measured by how hard or fast you push yourself, but by how well you listen to your body and respond to its needs.

Additionally, don't be afraid to take rest days or incorporate active recovery activities into your routine to give your joints a break and allow them to recover fully. Activities such as gentle stretching, foam rolling, or swimming can help alleviate stiffness and soreness while promoting joint health and mobility.

Tailoring Intensity and Duration

Embarking on a fitness journey as an endomorph woman is a journey of self-discovery and empowerment. With a body type that may require unique considerations when it comes to exercise intensity and duration, it's important to approach workouts with intention and mindfulness. Join me as we explore how to tailor intensity and duration to meet the needs of endomorph women, empowering you to achieve your fitness goals with confidence and grace.

Understanding Endomorph Women: Embracing Your Unique Physiology

Before delving into the specifics of intensity and duration, it's important to understand what sets endomorph women apart. Endomorph women typically have a higher body fat percentage and a tendency to store fat in areas such as the hips, thighs, and abdomen. Additionally, they may have a slower metabolism and reduced insulin sensitivity, which can impact energy levels and exercise performance.

Intensity Matters: Finding the Right Balance

When it comes to intensity, endomorph women may need to strike a delicate balance between pushing themselves enough to see results and avoiding overexertion that could lead to burnout or injury. High-intensity workouts can be effective for burning calories and improving cardiovascular health, but they may also be too taxing on the body, particularly for those with larger body sizes or joint issues.

Instead, consider incorporating a mix of moderate-intensity and high-intensity workouts into your routine. This allows you to challenge your body and push your limits without pushing too hard. Listen to your body's signals and adjust your intensity level as needed, focusing on feeling challenged but not overwhelmed during your workouts.

Duration: Quality Over Quantity

When it comes to workout duration, endomorph women may benefit from focusing on quality over quantity. Instead of long, grueling workouts that leave you feeling drained and exhausted, aim for shorter, more focused sessions that allow you to maximize your effort and intensity. High-intensity interval training (HIIT) can be particularly effective for endomorph women, as it allows you to achieve a high calorie burn in a shorter amount of time.

Additionally, consider incorporating rest periods into your workouts to allow your body to recover and recharge. This not only prevents overtraining and burnout but also allows you to maintain consistency in your workouts over the long term.

Mindful Movement: Listening to Your Body

Above all, it's essential for endomorph women to approach exercise with mindfulness and self-compassion. Pay attention to how your body feels during and after workouts, and honor its signals and limitations with kindness and grace. If something doesn't feel right, don't push through the pain; instead, modify the exercise or seek guidance from a qualified fitness professional.

Remember that progress is not measured by how hard or long you work out, but by how well you listen to your body and respond to its needs. By tailoring intensity and duration to meet the unique needs of your body, you can achieve your fitness goals in a way that feels sustainable and empowering.

CHAPTER 5
SAMPLE HIIT WORKOUTS FOR ENDOMORPH WOMEN

Beginner Level Workouts

People with an endomorph body type tend to have a slower metabolism, which makes it easier to gain weight and more challenging to lose weight. Exercise, especially cardiovascular exercise, is an important part in helping endomorphs burn more calories, increase metabolism, and lose weight. This means cardio is a key part of the endomorph workout plan.

So it's important that you do a cardio workout you love and have fun doing. Cardio not only helps you to achieve the health, fitness, and body goals you want, but also to maintain it.

Below are tips for choosing an exercise activity that you'll find comfortable and will enjoy, but is sufficiently intense to stimulate fat burning and weight loss

ENDOMORPH WORKOUT.

The ideal activity for endomorphs should be one that allows you to workout

- for at least 20 minutes
- engages the large muscle groups (e.g. legs, back)
- requires continuous, rhythmical movement (i.e. not stop and start like tennis)

- at moderate intensity or high intensity. Another factor to consider is how much impact an exercise has:
- Joint problems, previous injury, muscle imbalances and higher body weight increase the pressure on joints and bones during high-impact exercise, increasing the risk of injury.
- The more you weigh; the more force your body has to absorb.
- Body fat, bone and muscle mass all contribute to overall weight.

High-impact exercise is absolutely fine for endomorphs, but will be challenging if you have been sedentary or overweight. High-impact exercise (e.g. running) requires greater levels of fitness and strength to lift yourself off the ground, withstand the bigger impact and avoid injury. The more you weigh or the more out of shape you are, the tougher it gets. That means it's harder to exercise long enough (i.e. more than 20 minutes) to burn a significant amount of calories and that your risk of injury is greater.

That doesn't mean you shouldn't run, jump-rope or do any other high-impact workout. But just that if you're a beginner, you need to ease into it. Remember. Do what you love!

And whatever you do, don't throw yourself into a high-intensity, hard-core workout on day 1, only to swear off ever exercising again! You want to love exercising. And to understand that if something didn't work out, why it didn't, what to do next, and that it doesn't mean you can't try again later when you're stronger, more fit and a lot more fierce!

In terms of intensity, beginners should start at moderate level of intensity. In other words, if you're cycling for example, don't start out by cycling as fast as you can. Instead, adopt a more measured intensity, which will also allow you to exercise for longer. At moderate intensity you are breathing through your mouth, but still just about able to carry on a normal conversation. As you become more fit, you can increase the difficulty.

You can also supplement the above core exercises with extra activities, which offer variety, fun and team interaction, but are less effective calorie-burners.

Here are some examples of beginner-level workouts suitable for endomorph women:

1. **Bodyweight Circuit:**
   - Squats: 2 sets of 10-12 repetitions

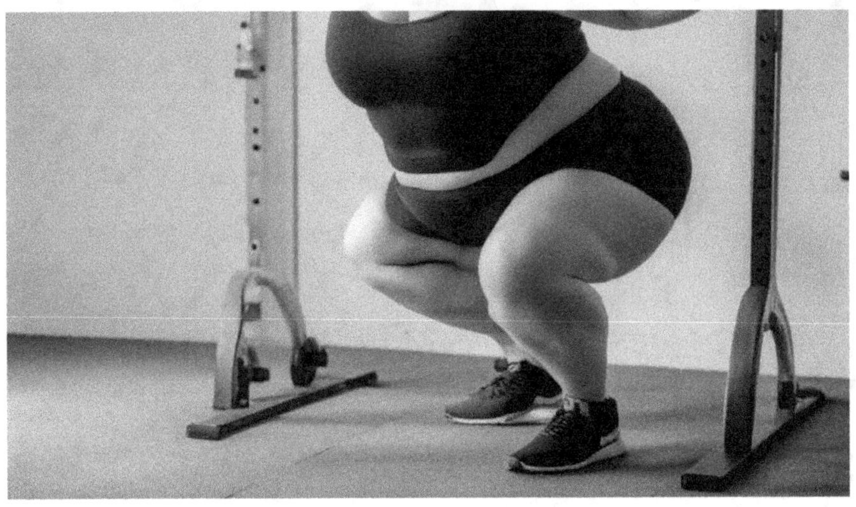

- Push-ups (on knees if needed): 2 sets of 8-10 repetitions

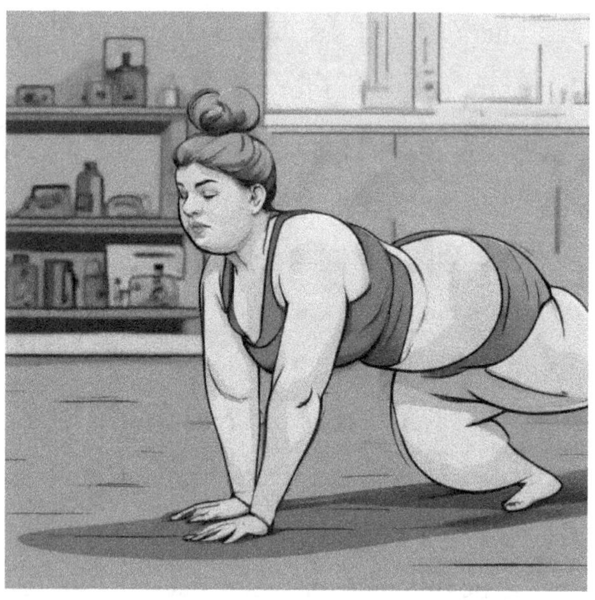

- Lunges: 2 sets of 10-12 repetitions per leg

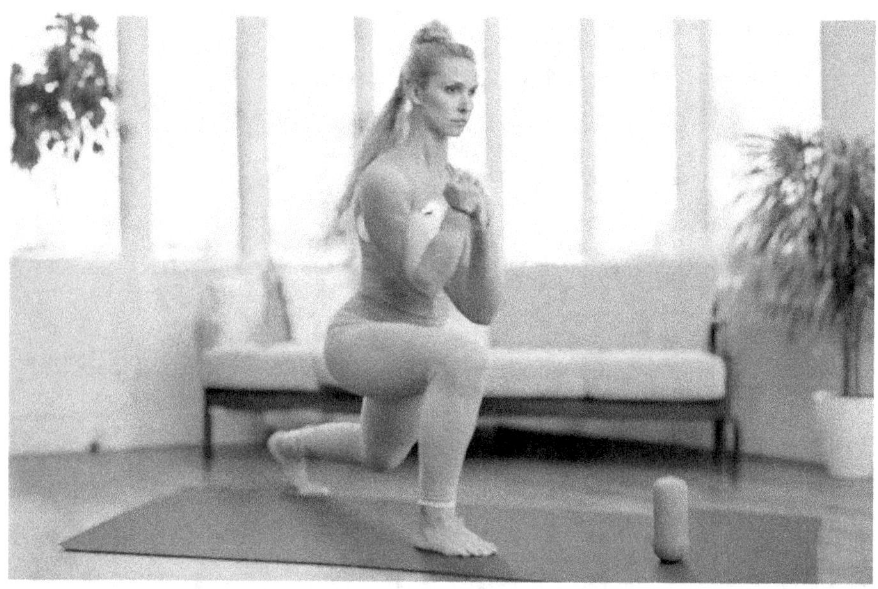

- Plank: Hold for 30 seconds to 1 minute

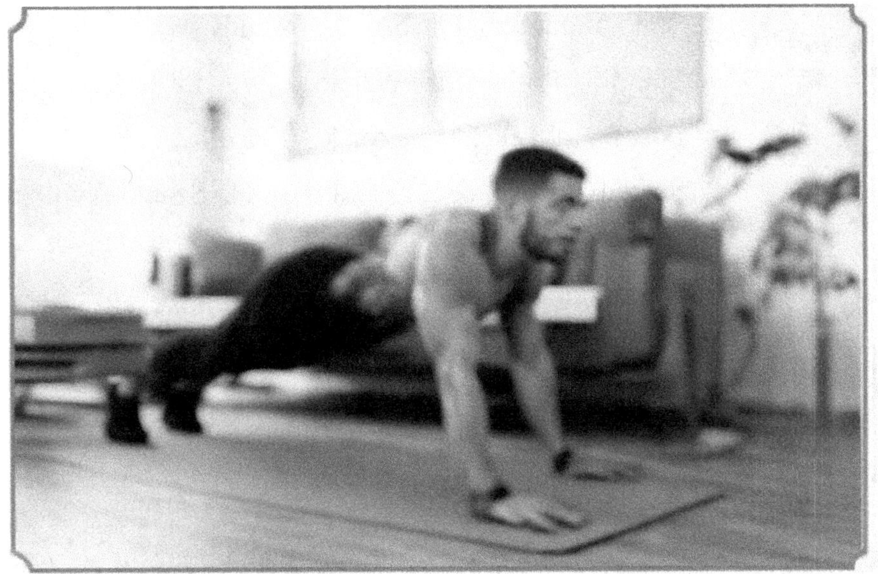

- Bodyweight Rows (using a sturdy table or low bar): 2 sets of 8-10 repetitions

2. **Walking Routine:**
   - Brisk walk around your neighborhood or local park: Start with 20-30 minutes and gradually increase to 45-60 minutes.
   - Aim for a pace where you can still hold a conversation but feel slightly breathless.

3. **Swimming Session:**
   - Swim laps at a leisurely pace for 20-30 minutes.
   - Focus on maintaining good form and breathing rhythm.

4. **Beginner Yoga Flow:**

   - Sun Salutations: Perform 2-3 rounds.

   - Standing Poses (e.g., Warrior I, Warrior II, Triangle Pose): Hold each pose for 5-10 breaths.

   - Seated Poses (e.g., Forward Fold, Seated Twist): Hold each pose for 5-10 breaths.

   - Cool Down with Savasana (Corpse Pose): Relax in Savasana for 5-10 minutes.

5. **Cycling Routine:**

   - Start with a 20-30 minute ride on flat terrain.

   - Gradually increase the duration and intensity as you become more comfortable.

6. **Elliptical Workout:**

   - Warm-up: 5 minutes at a moderate pace.

   - Main Workout: Alternate between 2 minutes of steady-state cardio and 1 minute of higher intensity intervals for 20-30 minutes.

   - Cool Down: 5 minutes at a comfortable pace.

Intermediate Level Workouts

Congratulations on reaching the intermediate level of your fitness journey! As an endomorph woman, progressing to this stage signifies your commitment to your health and well-being. Intermediate level workouts offer an opportunity to challenge your body, build strength, and continue making progress towards your fitness goals. Join me as we explore various types of exercises suitable for intermediate level workouts and how they can be carried out effectively to elevate your fitness routine.

Elevating Your Strength: Resistance Training

At the intermediate level, resistance training becomes even more important for building lean muscle mass, increasing metabolism, and improving overall strength and endurance. Incorporating a variety of compound exercises that target multiple muscle groups simultaneously is key to maximizing your results.

1. **Barbell Squats:** Perform 3-4 sets of 8-10 repetitions, focusing on maintaining proper form and depth.

2. **Deadlifts:** Complete 3-4 sets of 6-8 repetitions, ensuring a neutral spine and engaging your glutes and hamstrings.

3. **Bench Press:** Aim for 3-4 sets of 8-10 repetitions, with a focus on controlling the weight and engaging your chest and triceps.

4. **Pull-Ups or Assisted Pull-Ups:** Perform 3-4 sets of 6-8 repetitions, using an overhand grip to target your back muscles. As you progress, gradually increase the weight or resistance to continue challenging your muscles and stimulating growth. Remember to incorporate rest days into your routine to allow for proper recovery and muscle repair.

Revving Up Your Cardio: High-Intensity Interval Training (HIIT)

Intermediate level workouts often include high-intensity interval training (HIIT), which involves alternating between short bursts of intense exercise and brief periods of rest or lower-intensity activity. HIIT workouts are highly effective for burning calories, boosting metabolism, and improving cardiovascular fitness.

1. **Sprint Intervals:**

Warm up with 5-10 minutes of light cardio, then alternate between 30 seconds of sprinting and 60 seconds of walking or jogging for 20-30 minutes.

2. **Circuit Training:**

Perform a series of strength exercises (e.g., squats, lunges, push-ups) followed by short bursts of cardio (e.g., jumping jacks, mountain climbers) for 30-60 seconds each, with minimal rest between exercises. Complete 3-4 circuits.

HIIT workouts can be tailored to your fitness level and preferences, so feel free to experiment with different exercises and intervals to find what works best for you. Just be sure to listen to your body and modify the intensity as needed to avoid overexertion.

Balancing Mind and Body: Incorporating Yoga and Pilates

In addition to strength training and cardio, incorporating mindful practices such as yoga and Pilates into your routine can help improve flexibility, balance, and mental focus. These exercises also provide an opportunity to connect with your body and reduce stress, promoting overall well-being.

1. **Vinyasa Yoga Flow:**

Perform a series of flowing sequences that link breath with movement, focusing on building strength, flexibility, and endurance.

2. **Pilates Matwork:**

Engage in a series of Pilates exercises that target the core, hips, and shoulders, emphasizing proper alignment and controlled movements.

Both yoga and Pilates can be adapted to suit your fitness level, so don't hesitate to modify poses or use props as needed. Incorporate these practices into your routine 2-3 times per week to reap the full benefits.

Advanced Level Workouts

Welcome to the pinnacle of your fitness journey – the advanced level workouts. As an endomorph woman who has journeyed through beginner and intermediate stages, you have built a foundation of strength, endurance, and resilience. Now, it's time to elevate your workouts to new heights and challenge yourself in ways you never thought possible. Join me as we explore advanced level workouts, pushing the boundaries of what your body can achieve and unlocking your full potential.

1. Complex Compound Movements:

At the advanced level, compound movements become more complex and demanding, targeting multiple muscle groups simultaneously and promoting functional strength and athleticism.

- **Clean and Jerk:**

This Olympic weightlifting movement combines explosive power with precision technique. Start with a light weight and gradually increase as you become more proficient.

- **Snatch:**

Another Olympic lift that requires speed, coordination, and flexibility. Begin with a PVC pipe or light barbell to master the technique before adding weight.

- **Barbell Thrusters:**

Combining a front squat with an overhead press, thrusters are a full-body exercise that builds strength and power. Perform 3-4 sets of 6-8 repetitions with challenging weight.

2. Plyometric Training:

Plyometric exercises involve explosive movements that utilize the stretch reflex of muscles, improving power, speed, and agility.

- **Box Jumps:**

Start with a low box height and focus on landing softly with bent knees. As you become more proficient, gradually increase the height of the box to continue challenging yourself.

- **Plyo Push-Ups:**

Explosively push off the ground during the upward phase of the push-up, aiming to achieve maximum height with each repetition. Perform 3-4 sets of 8-10 repetitions.

- **Jump Squats:**

Descend into a squat position, then explode upwards into a jump, reaching maximum height before landing softly and immediately descending into the next squat. Complete 3-4 sets of 10-12 repetitions.

3. Advanced Cardiovascular Conditioning:

At the advanced level, cardiovascular workouts become more intense and challenging, pushing your limits and improving overall fitness levels.

- **Interval Sprints:**

Perform 30-second sprints at maximum effort, followed by 60 seconds of active recovery (walking or jogging). Repeat for 10-15 rounds.

- **Tabata Training:**

Alternate between 20 seconds of high-intensity exercise (e.g., burpees, mountain climbers) and 10 seconds of rest for 8 rounds. This protocol can be applied to a variety of exercises to create a challenging and effective workout.

- **Hill Sprints:**

Find a steep hill or set a treadmill to an incline and sprint uphill for 20-30 seconds, followed by a recovery walk or jog back down. Repeat for 8-10 rounds.

4. Advanced Core Strengthening:

At the advanced level, core exercises become more challenging and dynamic, targeting all muscles of the core for maximum strength and stability.

- **Hanging Leg Raises:**

Hang from a pull-up bar and lift your legs straight up towards the ceiling, engaging your lower abs. Lower with control and repeat for 3-4 sets of 10-12 repetitions.

- **Russian Twists with Medicine Ball:**

Sit on the floor with knees bent and feet off the ground, holding a medicine ball or weight. Rotate your torso from side to side, touching the ball to the floor on each side. Perform 3-4 sets of 12-15 repetitions per side.

- **Plank Variations:**

Challenge your core stability with advanced plank variations such as side planks, plank with leg lifts, or plank with arm reaches. Hold each variation for 30-60 seconds and repeat for 3-4 sets.

CHAPTER 6
RECOVERY AND NUTRITION STRATEGIES

Importance of Rest and Recovery

When our bodies repair, rebuild, and grow stronger, and our minds find solace and clarity amidst the chaos of daily life. Join me as we delve into the importance of rest and recovery, exploring how these vital components can elevate your fitness journey and nurture your body and mind.

1. Physical Restoration: Repairing the Body

Rest and recovery play a pivotal role in the physical restoration of our bodies, allowing muscles, joints, and tissues to heal and rebuild after the stresses of exercise. During intense workouts, our muscles undergo microscopic tears and breakdown, which, when properly rested, are repaired and strengthened, leading to muscle growth and increased strength.

2. Preventing Overtraining and Burnout: Finding Balance

In our eagerness to achieve our fitness goals, it can be tempting to push ourselves to the limit, training harder and longer in pursuit of progress. However, dear reader, there is a fine line between pushing ourselves to grow and pushing ourselves too far. Overtraining syndrome, characterized by persistent fatigue, decreased performance, and increased risk of injury, can derail even the most dedicated fitness journey.

3. Mental Rejuvenation: Nurturing the Mind

In addition to its physical benefits, rest and recovery are essential for mental rejuvenation and well-being. Regular rest allows our minds to unwind and recharge, reducing stress levels and promoting mental clarity and focus. Just as our bodies need time to repair and rebuild, so too do our minds need moments of stillness and calm amidst the chaos of daily life.

4. Maximizing Performance: The Power of Peaks and Valleys

Contrary to popular belief, dear reader, constant activity does not always lead to peak performance. In fact, it is during moments of rest and recovery that our bodies and minds are primed for optimal performance. By incorporating planned rest days and recovery periods into our workout regimens, we can ensure that we are always operating at our best, both physically and mentally.

5. Strategies for Effective Rest and Recovery: Nurturing Your Body and Mind

Now that we understand the importance of rest and recovery, let us explore some strategies for incorporating these vital components into our fitness routines:

- **Scheduled Rest Days:** Plan regular rest days into your workout schedule, allowing for both physical and mental recovery.

- **Active Recovery:** Engage in low-intensity activities such as walking, swimming, or yoga on rest days to promote blood flow and muscle recovery.

- **Quality Sleep:** Prioritize quality sleep by establishing a consistent sleep schedule, creating a relaxing bedtime routine, and ensuring a comfortable sleep environment.

- **Nutrition and Hydration:** Support your body's recovery efforts by fueling it with nutrient-dense foods and staying hydrated throughout the day.

6. Listening to Your Body: Honoring Your Needs

Above all, dear reader, listen to your body's signals and honor its needs. If you are feeling fatigued, sore, or run-down, it may be a sign that you need to prioritize rest and recovery. Trust in your body's wisdom and give yourself permission to rest without guilt or shame.

Nutritional Guidelines for Endomorph Women

As an endomorph woman embarking on your fitness journey, you understand that achieving your health and wellness goals requires more than just exercise – it also requires proper nutrition. But with so much conflicting information out there, it can be overwhelming to know where to begin. Fear not, for I am here to guide you through the nutritional guidelines specifically tailored to your endomorphic body type. Let us explore how you can nourish your body to support your fitness goals and achieve optimal health and vitality.

Understanding Your Endomorphic Body Type: The Foundation

Before we delve into nutritional guidelines, dear reader, let us first understand what it means to have an endomorphic body type. Endomorphs tend to have a naturally higher percentage of body fat and may struggle with weight loss or maintaining a lean physique. However, they also have the potential to build strong, shapely muscles with the right approach to nutrition and exercise.

1. Balance is Key: Macronutrient Distribution

When it comes to nutrition for endomorph women, balance is key. Aim to include a balance of macronutrients – carbohydrates, proteins, and fats – in each meal to support energy levels, muscle growth, and overall health.

- **Carbohydrates:** Focus on consuming complex carbohydrates such as whole grains, fruits, and vegetables, which provide sustained energy and fiber to keep you feeling full and satisfied.

- **Proteins:** Include lean sources of protein such as chicken, fish, tofu, beans, and lentils to support muscle repair and growth. Aim to include protein in each meal and snack throughout the day.

- **Fats:** Incorporate healthy fats from sources such as avocados, nuts, seeds, and olive oil to support hormone production, brain function, and satiety. Avoiding trans fats and excessive saturated fats is important for heart health.

2. Mindful Eating: Portion Control and Moderation

For endomorph women, portion control and moderation are essential components of a balanced diet. Pay attention to portion sizes and practice mindful eating to avoid overeating and unnecessary calorie consumption.

- **Listen to Your Body:** Eat when you're hungry and stop when you're satisfied. Avoid eating out of boredom or emotional cues, and tune in to your body's hunger and fullness signals.

- **Practice Portion Control:** Use smaller plates and bowls to help control portion sizes, and be mindful of serving sizes when dining out or preparing meals at home. Remember, it's not just what you eat but how much you eat that matters.

3. Hydration: The Unsung Hero of Nutrition

In addition to macronutrients, hydration plays a crucial role in supporting overall health and wellness for endomorph women. Aim to drink plenty of water throughout the day to stay hydrated and support proper digestion, metabolism, and cellular function.

- **Water is Key:** Aim to drink at least 8-10 glasses of water per day, or more if you're physically active or live in a hot climate. Carry a water bottle with you throughout the day to remind yourself to stay hydrated.

- **Hydrating Foods:** Incorporate hydrating foods such as fruits and vegetables into your diet, which contain high water content and can help contribute to your overall fluid intake.

4. Individualized Approach: Listen to Your Body

Dear reader, it's important to remember that nutritional guidelines are not one-size-fits-all. What works for one person may not work for another, so it's essential to listen to your body and find what works best for you.

- **Experiment and Adjust:** Pay attention to how different foods make you feel and adjust your diet accordingly. If you notice certain foods or eating patterns are affecting your energy levels or mood, consider making changes to support your overall well-being.

- **Seek Professional Guidance:** If you're unsure about where to start or need personalized guidance, consider seeking advice from a registered dietitian or nutritionist who can help create a tailored nutrition plan based on your individual needs and goals.

Hydration and Supplements

As you continue on your fitness journey as an endomorph woman, it's essential to pay close attention to your hydration levels and consider supplementing your diet with key nutrients to support your health and well-being. In this chapter, we will explore the importance of hydration and supplements specifically tailored to the needs of endomorph women, empowering you to make informed choices that nourish your body and support your fitness goals.

Hydration: The Foundation of Health

Hydration is the cornerstone of optimal health and wellness, dear reader. As an endomorph woman, staying adequately hydrated is especially crucial due to your body's tendency to retain water and potentially experience bloating and water retention. Let us delve into the importance of hydration and how you can ensure you're getting enough fluids throughout the day.

- **Water: Your Best Friend:** Water is essential for nearly every function in your body, from regulating body temperature to aiding digestion and nutrient absorption. Aim to drink at least 8-10 glasses of water per day, or more if you're physically active or live in a hot climate.

- **Hydrating Foods:** In addition to drinking water, incorporating hydrating foods such as fruits and vegetables into your diet can help contribute to your overall fluid intake. Foods like cucumbers, watermelon, and strawberries have high water content and can help keep you hydrated throughout the day.

- **Monitor Your Urine Color:** One easy way to gauge your hydration levels is to monitor the color of your urine. Aim for a pale yellow color, indicating that you're adequately hydrated. Dark yellow urine may be a sign that you need to drink more fluids.

Supplements for Endomorph Women: Navigating the Options
While a well-rounded diet should provide most of the nutrients your body needs, there are certain supplements that endomorph women may benefit from incorporating into their routine to support their health and fitness goals. Let's explore some key supplements to consider and how they can enhance your overall well-being.

- **Omega-3 Fatty Acids:** Omega-3 fatty acids, found in fatty fish like salmon, as well as fish oil supplements, have anti-inflammatory properties and may help reduce inflammation and support heart health. Consider adding a high-quality fish oil supplement to your daily routine.

- **Vitamin D:** Many people, especially those who live in northern climates or spend most of their time indoors, may be deficient in vitamin D. This essential nutrient plays a crucial role in bone health, immune function, and mood regulation. Consider taking a vitamin D supplement, especially during the winter months when sunlight exposure is limited.

- **Probiotics:** Probiotics are beneficial bacteria that support gut health and digestion. Endomorph women may benefit from taking a probiotic supplement to promote a healthy balance of gut bacteria and support digestion and nutrient absorption.

- **Multivitamin:** While it's always best to get nutrients from whole foods, a high-quality multivitamin can help fill in any gaps in your diet and ensure you're getting all the essential vitamins and minerals your body needs to thrive.

Consultation with a Healthcare Professional: Your Best Resource

Before starting any new supplement regimen, dear reader, it's important to consult with a healthcare professional to ensure it's safe and appropriate for your individual needs. A registered dietitian, nutritionist, or healthcare provider can help assess your current diet and lifestyle and make recommendations tailored to your specific goals and concerns.

CHAPTER 7
MONITORING PROGRESS AND ADJUSTING YOUR ROUTINE

Tracking Metrics and Measurements

The overall size and mass of the human body are used as proxy measures for many purposes for the assessment of health status, obesity, malnutrition, disease and work capacity. The measurements of different body parts which include the segmental lengths, bodily breadths, circumferences of the trunk and limbs and skin and subcutaneous tissue fold thicknesses are used for research and for designing the instruments and equipments for human use.

Measurement techniques need to be standardized so that different studies may become comparable.

A brief introduction of various instruments used for taking body measurements appears

below:

Weighing scales

There are two different types of weighing scales or weighing machines generally used. One is a

round disc on which the subject stands and the reading is taken directly from the scale which is

inset at the top of the weighing machine. Usually, weight up to the nearest 0.5 kg can be taken.

The other is a beam balance which is level actuated and the person stands on the platform and reading is taken after balancing the beam with appropriate weights. The calibration of this type of machine is much more precise and up to 50 gm can be measured.

Stadiometer

Stadiometer is used for measuring height and sitting height of the subjects. It comprises of a platform to which a rectangular vertical column is attached (Fig. 2.3). The subject has to stand against this column with his back touching it. A movable horizontal plate is attached to this vertical column which is brought down on the head of the subject. Alongside this movable plate, there is a counter from which the reading is taken directly.

Anthropometer rod

An anthropometer rod is generally 2 meter long. A single rod of such length can be very inconvenient to carry. Therefore it has been designed in the form of 4 inter-fitting rods of 50 cm each. The rods carry a Batch number specific for the instrument and another number which is similar for the inter-fitting edges of two segments of the rod. The rod is calibrated in centimeters and can measure up to a minimum value of 1 millimeter. A movable socket is also included which can be moved up or down for taking the measurements and it has a place for fitting a cross-bar. When the rod is held vertically the cross bar is in a horizontal position with which the top of the head is touched for the measurement of height.

The anthropometer has a fixed socket at the top in which another horizontal bar can be attached.

The top segment has two calibrations; one which increases upwards from the first segment and is used for reading the measurements and the other starts from the top. Two cross-bars can be fit each into each socket in the top segment of the anthropometer rod; one which is fixed at the top and the other which is movable. This forms a big caliper called "anthropometer compass" and is used for measuring major breadths and diameters of the body.

IBP/HA Body Measurements

One of the most important protocols of taking these measurements had been standardized by the International Biological Programme /Human Adaptability (IBP/HA) growth sub-committee in 1969 (Tanner et al. 1969, 1981). This protocol has immensely been used since then and innumerable studies are available which have utilized these recommendations. This is perhaps one of the best reasons why these recommendations find their place in this manual. The following is the list of measurements which have been standardized by the IBP/HA
growth sub-committee:

Gross Body Measurements

Body weight Stature/Supine length

Lengths or Heights of Body Parts

- Sitting height/Crown-rump length
- Suprasternal height
- Total arm length
- Upper arm length
- Forearm length
- Height of anterior superior iliac
- spine
- Height of tibiale
- Lower leg length
- Foot length
- Buttocks-knee length
- Head length
- Nose height
- Morphological face height
- Upper face height
- Ear length
- Head height

Diameters or Breadths of Body Parts

- Biacromial diameter
- Biiliocristal diameter
- Transverse chest
- Antero-posterior chest
- Head breadth

- Bizygomatic diameter
- Nose breadth
- Bigonial diameter
- Mouth width
- Lip thickness
- Minimum frontal diameter
- Ear breadth
- Bicondylar femur
- Bicondylar humerus
- Wrist breadth
- Hand breadth
- Ankle breadth

Circumferences or Girths of Body Parts

- Chest circumference
- Upper arm circumference (relaxed)
- Upper arm circumference (contracted)
- Calf circumference
- Thigh circumference
- Head circumference
- Neck circumference
- Abdominal circumference
- Forearm circumference
- Wrist circumference
- Ankle circumference

Skinfold Thickness

- Biceps

- Triceps

- Subscapular

- Suprailiac

- Forearm

- Thigh

- Medial calf

- Chest (juxta nipple)

- Midaxillary   Abdomen

As you embark on your fitness journey as an endomorph woman, it's essential to have a clear understanding of your progress and how your body is responding to your efforts. Tracking metrics and measurements can provide valuable insights into your health and fitness journey, empowering you to make informed decisions and stay motivated along the way. In this chapter, we will explore the importance of tracking metrics and measurements for endomorph women and how you can use this information to support your goals and celebrate your achievements.

Understanding Your Body: The Importance of Tracking

Tracking metrics and measurements is not just about numbers on a scale or inches lost – it's about gaining insight into how your body is responding to your workouts, nutrition, and lifestyle choices. By tracking key metrics over time, you can identify trends, set realistic goals, and make adjustments to your approach as needed.

1. Key Metrics to Track:

- **Body Weight:** While weight alone is not a perfect measure of health or fitness, tracking changes in body weight over time can provide valuable information about your progress. Aim to weigh yourself consistently, using the same scale and under the same conditions each time.

- **Body Measurements:** In addition to weight, tracking measurements such as waist circumference, hip circumference, and body fat percentage can provide a more comprehensive picture of your body composition and progress.

- **Fitness Performance:** Keep track of your fitness performance metrics, such as strength gains, endurance levels, and workout intensity. This could include tracking the number of repetitions you can perform, the amount of weight you can lift, or the duration and intensity of your cardio workouts.

- **Energy Levels and Mood:** Pay attention to how you feel on a day-to-day basis, including your energy levels, mood, and overall well-being. Tracking changes in energy levels and mood can help you identify patterns and make adjustments to your lifestyle to support your health and fitness goals.

2. Setting SMART Goals:

When it comes to tracking metrics and measurements, it's essential to set SMART goals – Specific, Measurable, Achievable, Relevant, and Time-bound. By setting clear and realistic goals, you can stay focused and motivated on your journey and celebrate your progress along the way.

- **Specific:** Define your goals with precision, focusing on what you want to achieve and why it's important to you.

- **Measurable:** Choose metrics that can be quantified and tracked over time, such as body weight, measurements, or fitness performance.

- **Achievable:** Set goals that are challenging but realistic based on your current fitness level, lifestyle, and resources.

- **Relevant:** Ensure that your goals align with your values, priorities, and long-term objectives.

- **Time-bound:** Establish a timeframe for achieving your goals, whether it's weeks, months, or years, and set deadlines to keep yourself accountable.

3. Celebrating Progress and Adjusting Course:

As you track your metrics and measurements over time, dear reader, remember to celebrate your progress and achievements, no matter how small. Each milestone reached is a testament to your dedication and hard work, and deserves to be celebrated.

- **Reflect on Your Journey:** Take time to reflect on how far you've come since you started your fitness journey, acknowledging the obstacles you've overcome and the progress you've made along the way.

- **Adjust Your Approach:** Use the insights gained from tracking metrics and measurements to make informed decisions and adjustments to your approach. If you're not seeing the progress you'd hoped for, consider making changes to your workout routine, nutrition plan, or lifestyle habits to better support your goals.

4. The Importance of Patience and Persistence:

Dear reader, it's important to remember that progress takes time, and transformation is a journey, not a destination. Be patient with yourself and trust in the process, knowing that every step forward, no matter how small, is bringing you closer to your goals.

Listening to Your Body

For endomorph women, tuning into the body's signals is not just beneficial; it's essential for achieving and maintaining optimal health. This chapter delves into the profound practice of body listening, tailored specifically for endomorph women, guiding you through understanding and responding to your body's unique needs.

Understanding Your Body's Language

Every body communicates, but not all of us understand the language. For endomorph women, who often experience distinct physiological patterns like faster weight gain and difficulties in shedding excess fat, paying close attention to bodily cues is crucial. These signals can range from the clear-cut pangs of hunger to the subtle hints of hormonal shifts.

Recognizing Signals

Hunger and Fullness: The sensations of hunger and fullness are your body's way of communicating energy needs. An endomorph might find that her body signals hunger more frequently. It's important to differentiate between true hunger and emotional eating. The former is a straightforward signal that your body needs fuel, while the latter can be a response to stress, boredom, or other emotional cues.

Energy Fluctuations: As an endomorph, you may notice that your energy levels fluctuate more markedly throughout the day. Listening to these patterns can tell you when to engage in energy-demanding activities and when to take rest.

Stress and Relaxation Responses: Your body's stress responses are strong indicators of when you need to step back and care for your mental health. As stress can exacerbate weight retention in endomorphs, paying attention to and managing stress becomes doubly important.

Interpreting What You Hear

Listening is only the first step; interpreting these signals correctly and responding appropriately is what truly matters. For example, a sudden craving for sweets might not be a call for sugar but rather a need for energy, which could be addressed with a balanced snack that includes proteins and healthy fats.

Holistic Health Tracking

To effectively listen to your body, maintaining a holistic view of your health is beneficial. This means observing not just what you eat or how much you exercise, but also how you sleep, manage stress, and maintain social connections.

Journaling for Better Insights: Keeping a health diary can enhance your ability to listen to your body. Note down what you eat, your exercise routine, your emotional state, and other factors like sleep quality and duration. Over time, patterns will emerge that can guide you in making health decisions more attuned to your body's needs.

Learning from Feedback: Every body's response to changes in diet, exercise, or lifestyle is unique. When you try a new workout routine or change your eating patterns, observe how your body responds. Does your energy increase? Do you feel more satiated?

The feedback your body gives is invaluable in sculpting a lifestyle that truly fits.

Minding the Mind-Body Connection

As you deepen your practice of listening to your body, you'll find that the physical and mental are intricately linked. Emotional states can influence physical health, and vice versa. For endomorph women, who often face stereotyping and body shaming, nurturing a positive body image is part of listening to and caring for your body.

Meditation and Mindfulness: These practices can enhance your capacity to listen to your body. Through mindfulness, you can develop a greater awareness of your bodily sensations and emotional states, helping you respond to your body's needs with greater sensitivity.

Yoga and Gentle Movement: These physical practices are excellent for endomorphs, providing a way to improve flexibility, strength, and cardiovascular health, while also offering an opportunity to tune into the body's needs and limits.

Adjusting Intensity and Frequency

For endomorph women, who may find that their bodies respond differently to exercise compared to other body types, the challenge lies in adjusting the intensity and frequency of workouts to optimize results and sustain motivation. This chapter explores how endomorph women can fine-tune their exercise regimens to align perfectly with their unique physiological traits.

Understanding the Endomorph Body Type

Endomorphs are characterized by a higher proportion of body fat and less muscle mass, which can influence metabolism and energy storage. This body type can make losing weight more challenging but not unachievable. It requires a strategic approach that considers how endomorph bodies metabolize food and respond to different types of exercise.

Customizing Your Exercise Intensity

Start with Moderate Intensity: High-intensity workouts can be effective for quick calorie burn, but they might also lead to quicker burnout or injury if not approached carefully. For endomorph women, starting with moderate-intensity exercises can help the body adjust without overwhelming it. Activities like brisk walking, gentle cycling, or water aerobics are excellent for building up endurance and fitness levels.

Gradually Increase Intensity: Once you are comfortable with moderate exercises, gradually increasing the intensity can help prevent plateaus and improve metabolic rate. Incorporating high-intensity interval training (HIIT) can be beneficial. However, it should be tailored to your current fitness level and increased gradually to monitor how your body responds.

Strength Training Is Key: Muscle mass naturally boosts metabolism, which is beneficial for endomorphs. Incorporating strength training into your routine two to three times a week can help build lean muscle. Focusing on large muscle groups through exercises like squats, deadlifts, and bench presses can be particularly effective.

Adjusting Exercise Frequency

Consistency Over Frequency: For endomorph women, how often you exercise might be less important than how consistently you do it. Three to five times a week can be ideal, but it's crucial to listen to your body and adjust as needed. It's about finding a rhythm that keeps you engaged without leading to exhaustion.

Rest and Recovery: Unlike what many intense workout regimens suggest, more is not always better, especially for endomorphs. Adequate rest days are essential not only for muscle recovery but also to prevent metabolic burnout. This can mean incorporating active recovery days, where you engage in light activities like stretching or yoga instead of full rest.

Balancing Cardio and Strength: While cardio is important for burning calories, it should be balanced with strength training to enhance metabolism and improve body composition. This balance will look different for each individual; some may benefit from more strength training while others might need focused cardio. The key is to adjust based on your progress and how your body feels.

Reflective Practice for Long-term Success

Monitor and Modify: Keep a detailed exercise log and review it regularly. Are you seeing improvements? How do you feel after increasing intensity? Adjusting your regimen based on these observations is crucial for continued progress.

Seek Professional Guidance: Working with a fitness coach who understands the endomorph body type can provide tailored advice and modifications based on personal progress and challenges.

Embrace Flexibility: Your body's needs can change over time—due to age, hormonal changes, or lifestyle adjustments. Remaining flexible in your approach allows you to adapt your routine to continue benefiting from your efforts.

Adjusting the intensity and frequency of workouts for endomorph women is not about adhering to a strict regimen but about embracing a flexible, reflective approach that respects the body's responses and needs. It's about crafting a personalized path to health that fosters not only physical strength but also a deep, enduring resilience and well-being.

CHAPTER 8
OVERCOMING CHALLENGES AND STAYING MOTIVATED

Dealing with Plateaus

This chapter seeks to unpack the phenomenon of plateaus, offering strategic insights and empathetic guidance tailored specifically for endomorph women, emphasizing a journey that values progress over perfection.

Understanding the Plateau

A plateau occurs when you no longer see progress despite continuing with your exercise and diet regimen. This is a common experience in weight loss and fitness journeys and can be incredibly frustrating. However, it's also a natural part of the body's adaptation process. For endomorph women, whose metabolic rates might naturally be slower, plateaus can seem more frequent and stubborn. Recognizing a plateau is the first step in overcoming it.

The Role of Metabolism

Endomorphs typically have a slower metabolism, which means their bodies are more efficient at storing nutrients and less efficient at burning them off. When progress stalls, it's often because the body has adapted to the current level of physical activity and caloric intake. This adaptation is your body's way of maintaining equilibrium, but it can be countered with the right strategies.

Strategies to Overcome Plateaus

Reassess Your Caloric Intake: As you lose weight, your body requires fewer calories to function than it did at a heavier weight. Recalculating your caloric needs to reflect your current weight can provide a clearer guideline for how much you should be eating.

Vary Your Exercise Routine: If your workout has become routine, so has your body's response to it. Mixing up your exercises not only reignites physical engagement but also mental interest. Incorporating different types of cardiovascular exercises and alternating your strength training routine can challenge your muscles and reignite progress.

Increase Muscle Mass: Since muscle tissue burns more calories than fat tissue, increasing your muscle mass can help elevate your resting metabolic rate. Integrating more strength training into your routine can be effective. Focus on compound movements that target multiple muscle groups, which can be more beneficial than isolation exercises.

Enhance Exercise Intensity: Sometimes, increasing the intensity of your workouts can help break through a plateau. This might mean adding interval training to your routine or increasing the weights you lift. It's essential to do this gradually to avoid injury and to monitor how your body responds to these changes.

Psychological and Emotional Considerations

Stay Motivated: Plateaus can be mentally exhausting. Setting small, achievable goals can help maintain motivation during these times. Celebrate other signs of progress, like improved endurance, strength, or how your clothes fit, rather than just the number on the scale.

Manage Stress: High stress levels can lead to hormonal imbalances that might contribute to weight stagnation. Practices such as yoga, meditation, or simply taking time to unwind and relax can be integral in managing stress and aiding overall progress.

Seek Support: Connecting with others who are also navigating the challenges of fitness can provide encouragement, share strategies, and reduce feelings of isolation. Whether it's a community online or a local group, support networks can be invaluable.

Reflect and Adjust

Regularly Review Your Plan: Every few weeks, take time to review and adjust your fitness and diet plan. This regular audit allows you to stay proactive and flexible in your approach to overcoming plateaus.

Consult Professionals: Sometimes, an outside perspective can be crucial. A dietitian or a personal trainer who understands the unique needs of endomorph body types can offer personalized advice and adjustments that might be needed to move past a plateau.

For endomorph women, dealing with plateaus is part of the journey towards achieving and maintaining health and fitness goals. It's a sign that your body is adapting and requires new challenges and adjustments. By embracing plateaus as opportunities for growth and learning, you transform what might seem like a roadblock into a stepping stone towards your wellness aspirations.

Managing Time and Energy Constraints

In a world that races against time, managing both time and energy efficiently becomes not just a necessity but a form of self-care and empowerment, especially for endomorph women. The unique physiological traits of the endomorph body type, characterized by a predisposition to store energy as fat, demand a nuanced approach to time and energy management. This chapter delves into strategies specifically tailored for endomorph women, aiming to help them harness their full potential by aligning their fitness and wellness goals with the realities of their busy lives.

Understanding the Endomorph Challenge

Endomorphs often experience a slower metabolism and a higher fat storage when compared to other body types. This intrinsic nature can influence energy levels throughout the day, affecting everything from workout intensity to motivational states. Recognizing how your body type influences your daily energy fluctuations is crucial in planning a manageable and effective schedule.

Strategic Time Management

Prioritize Your Activities: Time management is fundamentally about prioritizing. For endomorph women, it is essential to prioritize activities that promote a healthy metabolism and energy levels. This includes regular physical activity, adequate sleep, and stress management practices.

Create a Routine: Consistency can be a powerful tool for managing a slow metabolism. Setting a routine that includes specific times for meals, exercise, and relaxation can help regulate your body's internal clock and improve metabolic efficiency.

Be Realistic: Set achievable goals within reasonable time frames. Overcommitting can lead to stress and burnout, which can be particularly detrimental for endomorphs as stress can exacerbate weight retention.

Energy Optimization Techniques

Balanced Nutrition: For endomorph women, managing energy is not just about managing time but also about managing how food converts to energy. A diet focused on a balanced intake of proteins, fats, and low-glycemic carbohydrates can help maintain steady energy levels throughout the day.

Incorporate Short, Intense Workouts: Given time constraints, short bouts of high-intensity interval training (HIIT) can be particularly effective. HIIT sessions can boost metabolism in a shorter period, making them ideal for those with busy schedules.

Active Breaks: Integrating short active breaks into the day can boost energy levels and counteract the metabolic slowdown associated with the endomorph body type. Even a few minutes of stretching or walking can make a significant difference.

Psychological Strategies for Energy Management

Mindfulness and Mental Framing: Psychological resilience plays a vital role in how energy is perceived and utilized. Mindfulness can help manage stress and improve mental clarity, making it easier to tackle daily tasks energetically.

Visualization Techniques: Visualizing daily goals and achievements can provide motivational boosts. This technique helps in reinforcing the belief that time and energy management are within one's control, despite physiological challenges.

Cognitive Reframing: Shift the narrative from viewing your body type as a limitation to seeing it as a unique aspect of your identity that you can manage and optimize. This mindset shift can significantly impact how you manage energy and approach your day.

Tailoring Approaches to Individual Lifestyles

Single Tasking versus Multitasking: While multitasking may seem like an efficient use of time, it can lead to decreased quality and increased stress. Focus on single tasks where possible to maximize efficiency and reduce overwhelm.

Technology as a Tool: Use technology wisely—employ apps and devices that help track fitness, nutrition, and time management. Set reminders for workouts, breaks, and meal times to keep on track without feeling overwhelmed.

Community Engagement: Sometimes, sharing the journey can ease the load. Engaging with a community of like-minded individuals or other endomorph women can provide emotional support, practical advice, and motivational boosts.

Finding Support and Accountability

For many endomorph women, weight management and achieving fitness goals can often feel like a solitary battle. However, incorporating a layer of social support and accountability can not only ease this journey but also enhance the outcomes. Studies have consistently shown that individuals who engage in health and fitness regimes with support from others tend to stick to their routines more consistently and are generally more successful in achieving their goals.

Identifying Your Needs

Before seeking out or building a support network, it's crucial for endomorph women to define what kind of support they need. Do they require emotional encouragement, practical tips for diet and exercise, or someone to physically accompany them on their workouts? Understanding these needs helps in targeting the right sources of support and structuring the type of accountability that will be most effective.

Sources of Support

Fitness Communities and Groups: Many communities focus specifically on fitness and health, with some tailored towards women with endomorph body types. Joining such groups can provide not only companionship and moral support but also valuable insights into what works for others with similar physiological traits.

Professional Guidance: Engaging with fitness trainers and nutritionists who understand the endomorph body type can transform a generic fitness plan into a personalized and effective regime. These professionals not only provide accountability but can also adjust dietary and exercise plans based on progress and feedback.

Digital Platforms: In today's digital age, a plethora of apps and online communities offer virtual companionship and accountability. These platforms can be particularly useful for those who may not have

CONCLUSION

Embarking on a fitness journey as an endomorph woman comes with its unique challenges, but remember, it's also an empowering path to self-discovery and health. Over the course of this guide, we've explored various strategies tailored specifically to your body type, from beginner workouts to HIIT protocols designed just for you. Now, as we draw these discussions to a close, it's time to reflect on what we've learned and how you can carry forward with momentum and motivation.

You are not alone in feeling that sometimes the mountain seems too steep, or progress too slow. Every step you take towards your fitness goals is a step towards a healthier, more vibrant you. The insights we've shared are not just guidelines but tools for you to reshape and reclaim your health, in a way that honors your body's natural tendencies and strengths.

The journey of health and fitness for an endomorph woman is not just about losing weight or building stamina; it's about creating a lifestyle that amplifies your wellbeing. It's about finding balance in your workouts, your diet, and your recovery periods. It's about adjusting intensity and frequency of exercises as your body speaks to you, telling you what it needs at different stages of your fitness journey.

Your path will have ups and downs. Some days will be tougher, requiring more from you, and it's okay to acknowledge this. Remember, every workout doesn't need to be perfect, and every day doesn't need to end in exhaustion. Balance is key, and rest is just as important as activity. Learning to listen to your body and understanding the signs it gives you is crucial. This communication is your greatest guide.

As you move forward, keep in mind that consistency is more transformative than intensity. Small, daily actions lead to significant changes over time. Build routines that fit into your life realistically and sustainably. Use the support systems we discussed to maintain motivation and accountability. Whether it's a community, a workout partner, or a coach, find your tribe that cheers you on and holds you accountable.

Moreover, don't underestimate the power of your own mindset. Cultivate a positive, forgiving attitude towards yourself and your progress. Celebrate every victory, no matter how small. These celebrations build your confidence and reinforce your commitment to your fitness journey.

In moments of doubt or frustration, remember why you started. Recall the vision of health you want to achieve and let that vision pull you forward. Keep pushing, keep striving, and keep evolving. Your goals are not just dreams; they are the blueprint for your continued efforts.

Lastly, I want to leave you with a quote that encapsulates the spirit of your journey:

"Strength does not come from physical capacity. It comes from an indomitable will." - Mahatma Gandhi

This quote isn't just about the strength needed to complete another set or run another mile; it's about the mental and emotional strength to persevere through challenges, to get up when you fall, and to keep going even when the finish line seems far away. Your will—your determination to keep moving forward—is your greatest strength.

Harness it, nurture it, and let it propel you through each step of your fitness journey. You are capable of amazing transformations, and your path as an endomorph woman is uniquely yours to shape. Shine in your resilience and let your journey be a beacon of encouragement not only to yourself but also to those around you who may be fighting their own battles.

Here's to stepping into your power each day with determination and grace, towards a healthier, happier you.

www.ingramcontent.com/pod-product-compliance
Lightning Source LLC
Chambersburg PA
CBHW050822250726
48653CB00006B/2373